GW00468340

[Iconographia]

a Franco Maria Ricci edition

FASHION IN PARIS

from the 'Journal des Dames et des Modes'
1912 - 1913

Introduction by
Cristina Nuzzi

Thames and Hudson

Translated from the Italian and the French by John Shepley

Any copy of this book issued by the publisher as a paperback is sold subject to the condition that it shall not by way of trade or otherwise be lent, re-sold, hired out or otherwise circulated, without the publisher's prior consent, in any form of binding other than that in which it is published and without a similar condition including these words being imposed on a subsequent purchaser.

© 1980 by Franco Maria Ricci, Milan, and Thames and Hudson, London

All rights reserved. No part of this publication may be reproduced or transmitted in any form or by any means, electronic or mechanical, including photocopy, recording, or any information storage or retrieval system, without permission in writing from the publisher.

Designed by Franco Maria Ricci
Edited by Laura Casalis
Colour separations by Zincografica Vaccari, Modena
Text composed in Bodoni Italics
Printed in Italy by GEA S.p.A., June 1980

Introduction

The year 1912 saw the emergence in the fashion world of three important magazines, expressions of the most refined Parisian elegance, and illustrated by the most gifted designers and illustrators of the time: La Gazette du Bon Ton, *founded and published by Lucien Vogel;* Modes et Manières d'Aujourd'hui, *issued by Corrard and Meynial; and* Le Journal des Dames et des Modes. *All three echoed in their titles publications that had appeared in the eighteenth and nineteenth centuries.*
The Journal des Dames et des Modes *lasted only two years (the first issue appeared on 1 June 1912, and the last on 1 August 1914). This stylish periodical was issued regularly three times a month, and ceased publication upon the outbreak of the First World War. With its expensive layout, its society columns, its poetic texts, its colourful annotations, and its fashion reports, it represented the last brilliant, refined, impartial, and aestheticizing impulse of a happy and optimistic society occupying the centre of the stage in the period that has aptly been called the 'belle époque'.*
As an organ of fashion, the Journal, *in its title and recherché appearance, was following in the footsteps (same type, same paper and format) of a successful nineteenth-century periodical, famous for its plates of 'Costumes Parisiens', which had been started in 1798 by an enterprising abbé, Pierre de La Mésangère, and continued to appear until 1839. Like its model, the new magazine was not simply a fashion vehicle. It was essentially the testimony, the history - illustrated, or rather 'clothed' and narrated - of the customs, ideas, and ideals of a society and a period. It was founded by a 'personality' of the time: Tom Antongini, secretary and friend of Gabriele D'Annunzio, and himself a writer, who had followed the poet into his Parisian exile. Antongini later described his publishing venture as follows:*
'From February 1912 on, I only went to Arcachon a couple of times a month, and only when the Poet did not come to Paris in person. Paris was now my permanent residence, because of a publishing enterprise I had undertaken, with the initial support of the Poet himself. I had already set up a company for the publication of a fashion journal, designed for lovers of rare editions, printed in 1,250 copies, with copperplate illustrations successively coloured by stencils. It was called Journal des Dames et des Modes, *and represented the continuation of a celebrated journal that had first appeared towards the end of the eighteenth century.... Joining me as co-editor in this attempt at artistic resurrection was a certain Jacques de Nouvion, a cultivated and experienced journalist, of extraordinary graciousness, whom I had previously had the opportunity to introduce to the Poet when matters were still in the planning stages.... D'Annunzio not only subscribed to our publication but was generous in giving me letters of recommendation and moral support. He took a great interest in it... and it was solely thanks to him that I was able to count from the first issue on the highly desired collaboration of Anatole France, Madame de Noailles, and other famous French writers of the time.'*
The magazine thus got off to an auspicious start: born in a refined cultural and intellectual atmosphere and designed to appeal to an audience of aesthetes, it sought to distinguish itself from such already existing periodicals in this field as Fémina *or* La Vie Parisienne. *Anatole France, at D'Annunzio's personal solicitation, acted as godfather and wrote an introduction for the first issue, in which he explained the magazine's intentions and stressed its historical usefulness:*

'Some fifteen years ago one could still find on the shelves of second-hand booksellers or at print dealers a few scattered volumes and loose prints of the Journal des Dames et des Modes, published from Year V until 1839, and which among connoisseurs and booksellers was known simply as La Mésangère. Nowadays the complete set is unobtainable and the smallest remnants fetch very high prices.

'I do not know whether serious people sometimes scorned La Mésangère; serious people are frequently a little foolish. But of one thing I am certain, and that is that La Mésangère is a precious monument of French history at the end of the eighteenth century and the beginning of the nineteenth. One knows nothing of a society when one knows nothing of the fashions that prevailed in it. Costumes reveal customs, and the toilettes of Citizenesses Tallien and Beauharnais, for example, can help us to understand the spirit of Thermidor. The historian of the Revolution or the Empire who has not spent a good deal of time perusing the fashion journals is, to my mind, extremely limited.

'La Mésangère is not the oldest of these journals, but it offers the uninterrupted sequence of French fashions for forty-one years. And it does so in 3,624 engraved colourplates, each of which is a little masterpiece. These plates are for the most part the work of Debucourt and Horace Vernet; collectors today vie for them eagerly.

'Nor is the text of the Journal des Dames et des Modes lacking in interest. There one can find curious anecdotes about the society that smilingly witnessed so many revolutions. This charming journal disappeared in 1839, absorbed by a later publication, Le Follet. We do not know what led to its end. Perhaps the death of La Mésangère, who was the soul of these delightful little issues. Moreover, the age was now a very romantic, as well as a very industrial one; the tradition of engraving and of good typography was in decline; the Journal des Dames et des Modes could not have preserved its old-fashioned charm with the invasion of cheap printing. It had done well to die.

'Seventy-five years later it is being reborn. It is being reborn through the efforts of a few artists and talented spirits.

'It is being reborn for connoisseurs (if there are any left) who are not satisfied with fashion journals that have a circulation of several thousand copies and are illustrated by photography. And if the publishers are bringing back to us, with exactly the same format, paper, printing, and engraving and colour techniques, the old classic of fashion from former times, it is because they intend it to continue pleasantly and become the delightful fashion classic of today and tomorrow.'

In addition to Anatole France's influential presence, the first issue of the magazine (printed in an edition of 1,250 copies on Holland paper, plus 29 deluxe copies on Japan paper) contained other exceptional contributions. There were Parnassian verses by the Comtesse Anna de Noailles (1876-1933), the poetess who was also a muse of the period. She customarily received her friends, who included the most outstanding poets and intellectuals, from Anatole France to Gide and Colette, while reclining on a divan amid luxurious fabrics and objets d'art; Proust called her 'a Carthaginian goddess who inspired ideas of lust in everyone'. Next came a facetious set of rules for the drawing-room conversationalist, drawn up with subtle irony by Henri Duvernois (1875-1937), already a well-known novelist and playwright but destined to achieve still greater fame later on. Paul Reboux reviewed the Paris theatre, from Jean Moréas's Iphigénie to the Ballets Russes. Diaghilev's company had just offered two new works, Le Dieu Bleu and Thamar, danced by Bolm, Karsavina, and Nijinsky, and with music by Hahn and Balakirev respectively, barbaric, Oriental dances and bold-coloured sets and costumes by Léon Bakst.

After a few ironic observations by Marcel Boulenger on the advantages of retiring to the country, the issue closed with some notes on fashion: stylish men no longer wear a flower in the buttonhole of an evening suit; in the morning ladies are wearing white woollen or flannel tailormades; the crinoline is going out of fashion, there is an obvious trend toward flowing lines and drapery. Detailed information is illustrated by references to particular places and occasions. For example:

'Robes de lingerie *have already been seen at Auteuil and Longchamp, many of them trimmed with lace and adorned with tucks of black silk muslin in the lace. The black velvet trimming that was all the rage last year will not be seen again this year. So much the better! But the black silk muslin is also too much. For trimming our* robes de lingerie, *a few small pieces of fine lace should always be sufficient, with a large rose of France on the bodice.'*

The issue was completed with three colour engravings, one reproducing a fashion plate printed a century earlier on the cover of La Mésangère. The other two plates were the work of two young designers, Bernard Boutet de Monvel (1881-1949) and Georges Barbier (1882-1932), of whom more later. The Journal *did not scorn advertising, and in each issue, consisting of sixteen pages, four were reserved for the austerely stylish publicizing of prestigious fashion houses and suppliers. Thus, on the subject of perfumes, we learn that the year's new products from the Maison Guerlain are called 'Vague Souvenir', 'Pour troubler', and 'Kadine', and that the Edizioni Musicali Lorenzo Sonzogno will shortly publish Gabriele D'Annunzio's* Fedra, *with music by Ildebrando Pizzetti, as well as a new tragedy by the same poet entitled* Parisina, *with music by Pietro Mascagni.*

Striking innovations had already transformed the fashion scene at the time the Journal des Dames et des Modes *appeared. The revolution which had been* brought about by Paul Poiret (d. 1944) had drawn its inspiration from the creations of the Russian designers for Diaghilev's company.

Inspired by the Persian and Indian Orient, Poiret abolished corsets and stays, creating clothing with soft and supple lines that followed the natural contours of the body. These designs had been skillfully illustrated and publicized in 1908 by Paul Iribe (Les robes de Paul Poiret racontées par Paul Iribe) *and in 1911 by Georges Lepape* (Les choses de Paul Poiret), *and later achieved a kind of official stamp in the famous costume ball entitled 'La Mille et Deuxième Nuit' or 'Persian Celebration', given by Poiret and attended by* le Tout Paris.

Though the Parisian fashion world in the years 1910-12 displayed a variety of trends and influences (such as a revival of eighteenth-century fashions and neoclassical elements), it was the Oriental inspiration which triumphed, as we can see from plates published in 1912 in the Christmas Issue of Fémina. *These were the work of Barbier, Brunelleschi, Manuel Orazi and Lepape, and represented, respectively, 'La Comédie française', 'La Comédie italienne', 'La Comédie anglaise', and 'La Comédie persane', a confrontation which led to the palm being accorded to the 'Persian' style. As Henry de Régnier wrote in his article 'La mode, la femme et la Perse', 'It was the period of ottomans and sofas, of babouches and turbans...'*

Though these years were dominated by the personality of Poiret, other couturiers helped to make Paris the major fashion centre of the West, the capital of elegance, to which the eyes of the rest of the world were turned.

Worth (one of the oldest fashion houses), and the firms of Madame Chéruit (to whom Poiret had brought his first sketches in 1898) and the Callot sisters in the rue Taitbout belonged to an older generation, but still showed signs of wishing to keep up with the new trends. Jacques Doucet (1853-1929), in his fashion house on the rue de la Paix, was still supplying his clientele with clothing of refined taste adorned with lace and similar expensive materials. It was with Doucet, the leading and most talented representative of the older generation, that the young Poiret had served his apprenticeship, before moving, with the help of his generous teacher, to the rue de l'Auber in 1903. Doucet, who had created clothes for Sarah Bernhardt and Réjane, was said to have sold his collection of eighteenth-century art in 1912 under the influence of Poiret, to replace it with works of modern art and African sculpture. In 1913, his model 'Le Coup de Vent', designed by Robert Dammy for the Gazette du Bon Ton showed that he had simplified his line while preserving his taste for expensive trimmings.

Alongside the established firms, new houses were springing up. There was Madame Jenny, who opened her atelier in 1909; Nicole Groult, formerly Poiret's assistant, who set herself up in the rue d'Anjou in 1910; and later Martial and Armand, Paquin, Beer and Rigaud.

Figures of greater talent and importance were Jeanne Lanvin (1867-1946), Gabrielle Bonheur, known as Coco Chanel (1883-1971), and Madeleine Vionnet (1878-1974). Lanvin, destined to dominate the Paris scene until her death, was originally a milliner. She took up haute couture around 1905, numbering among her clientele some of the most prominent names in the intellectual and theatrical worlds and the aristocracy. It was in one of her dresses that the Comtesse de Noailles chose to be buried. Coco Chanel, who was to have such an important influence on postwar fashion in creating the garçonne, the dynamic and active woman dressed in clothes with simple and comfortable lines, began her Paris career around 1909-10. Finally, Madeleine Vionnet, who had been an apprentice with Doucet and Chéruit, opened her first showroom in 1910, and became famous for her diagonal line. All

three, though at first influenced by Orientalism, later turned to more linear conceptions, drawing inspiration from the Cubist painting so strongly represented at the Salon des Indépendants in 1912.

Thus when the Journal made its first appearance, the fashion world contained a number of distinct personalities, and was in a state of ferment and expansion. The magazine did not fail to record in each of its issues all the changes that were then taking place, whether affecting dresses, hats, gloves, shoes, umbrellas, fans or jewelry. Observations, though detailed, usually did not mention the names of the couturiers. An exception was made on one occasion when Jeanne Lanvin attended the races at Longchamp boldly attired in one of her own creations. In No. 34 (1 May 1913), we read:

'Much remarked, at this same gathering, was Madame Jeanne Lanvin, who, in working costume – brown tailormade over which she had thrown a long mantle with collar wrapped around her neck like a democratic muffler, and her face hidden under a thick black veil – looked like a general inspecting the field before launching the attack. More and more our Parisian racecourses are branches of the showrooms of our great artists of dressmaking.'

But what is fashion? Lucie Delarue-Mardrus, the capricious writer so enamoured of everything Oriental that she liked to appear at costume parties on horseback dressed as an Arab chieftain, discussed the question in a piece appearing in No. 11 (10 September 1912), entitled 'Si la mode est un art?' Today her arguments may be questioned, but they express the thinking of the time.

'This question, so often asked, is quite surprising. For if fashion is not an art, then what is it?

'If it were simply a matter of clothing oneself, fashion would certainly not exist. But it is above all a matter of attiring oneself, and whoever says attire says ornament, and whoever says ornament says art....

'Fashion is noble, fashion is documentary. What else is it? It is something less serious and more sensitive: it is charming.

'It is especially while thinking of fashion – this ever-changing butterfly, fashion which creates a new being by adorning the same body, fashion which transforms silhouettes, fashion which dissolves or straightens lines, fashion, this art - this great art - it is especially while thinking of fashion that I marvel that women complain and wear themselves out in so-called 'feminist' demands.

'How can one think of feminism when there is femininity?...

'Certainly fashion is a more serious thing than is believed. To it go the honour and responsibility of adorning the crowd and for varying its image according to the times. One has heard much talk of uplifting the people through visits to museums. There is no more beautiful museum than the one in action, constituted by women passing in the street.

'So, ladies, be stylish. It is a great civic duty. Though Notre-Dame is a cathedral, it is nonetheless une dame. May your exterior be also the cathedral of your soul.

'I know, of course, that this cathedral sometimes turns to extravagance. And I am the first to wish to see the disappearance, for example, of those huge hats that make women look as if they were taking their tub-baths upside down. But I am not sorry to see that women push their preoccupation with fashion to the point of martyrdom.

'From crinoline to hobble skirts, from panniers to leg-of-mutton sleeves, from soaring coiffures to bustles and poufs, women, already so sorely tried by the ills of their nature, are capable, should fashion demand it, of undergoing the most refined tortures. They make themselves fatter here, thinner there, from being stretched to the utmost they go to the most monstrous breadth, and on this bed of Procrustes they smile: fashion is truly a garden of tortures. And yet, among so many female demands, there is not one woman who cries for help, not one hidden corset that revolts, not one pair of legs that breaks its fetters.....

'Yes, women, in order to follow fashion, are capable of heroism. After all, might it not be their way of going to war?

'Be that as it may, it is rather beautiful to think that fashion, which is the most vital of the arts, is also the most cruel, and that nevertheless its adepts increasingly multiply and will not stop multiplying as long as there are women on earth.'

In each issue, the magazine published precise fashion notes of practical interest to its women readers. In August 1912 (No. 8) one learns that:

'Slimness triumphs. Artificial or real, the slim woman is displaying her Tanagraean silhouette. It is a considerable phenomenon, which affects and will continue to affect, if this fashion lasts, the whole social equilibrium. But will it last? Why not? Everything concurs in it.' The next issue foresees the end of the Persian style: 'It is probably all over for Persian costume balls.... We will never again see this mad bedizenment, this eccentricity of forms, of colours, of hairdos, for which they were the artistic pretext'. The same issue points to the early appearance of furs: 'This year, we believe, furs have beaten the record for precocity. They made their appearance on 15 August on the Champs-Elysées; but they had already been displayed for several days in Trouville-Deauville and on many beaches.'

Nevertheless, though every issue carefully reviewed all the current novelties of fashion, the Journal did not cease to recommend to both its men and women readers that they adopt only those styles truly worthy of being called elegant.

Every issue carried coloured stencil prints reproducing the latest conceptions of the fashion designers.

The magazine also welcomed literary contributions. As we have seen, it was thanks to D'Annunzio that the magazine could count on the collaboration of the best known writers and littérateurs of the time. Among the most diligent – almost all the first year's issues contained a contribution by him – was Henri Duvernois. He supplied brilliant and witty observations on day-to-day life (theatre audiences, the passing parade), ironic advice for those hoping to frequent good society as well as chronicles of events – brief accounts written with veiled irony and subtle melancholy. Marcel Boulenger, journalist of the Figaro and contributor to many other publications, including La Vie Parisienne, contributed brilliant paragraphs depicting the society of the time, book reviews and witty comments on daily happenings. Other famous names to appear were the novelists Paul Margueritte (1860-1918), René Boyslesve (1867-1926), Henri Barbusse (1873-1935) - who was to win the Goncourt Prize in 1916 for his 'war diary' Le Feu - and Francis de Miomandre (b. 1880), the dramatists Pierre Veber (b. 1869) and Henri Lavedan (1859-1940), and the poets Fernand Gregh, Jean Cocteau and Paul Géraldy. No. 37 (1 June 1913) published an excerpt from La Pisanelle ou la Mort parfumée by D'Annunzio, staged shortly afterwards (12 June) at the Théatre Châtelet, with sets and costumes by Bakst, music by Pizzetti and performed by Ida Rubinstein. It was a resounding success.
Other frequent contributors were Fernand Vandérem and Pierre de Trévières, whose writings likewise often appeared in other publications of the period, from Fémina to the Gazette du Bon Ton. The Journal also published pieces by Pierre Mille, André Picard, secretary of the Exposition Universelle of 1900, Franc-Nohain, author of the libretto for L'Heure espagnole by Ravel, Roger Boutet de Monvel and others.
No less important were the artistic contributions which included the works of some outstanding artists and many promising young ones.
Most frequent in his appearance, and outstanding for the quality of his illustrations, was Georges Barbier, a young painter from Nantes. Barbier, who had recently emerged from the Ecole des Beaux-Arts, still seemed in his early works (pls. 3 and 8) to be somewhat restrained by his concern for 'pure' and precise design; thus he showed in the high-waisted Tailleur in Pearl-Grey Silk, recalling Empire models, that he had not yet responded to more advanced precepts of fashion. But in the Pink Damask Cloak Trimmed with Blue Fox (pl. 35), he revealed that he had mastered his style, not so much by adhering to the 'Persian taste', but by his richer and more dazzling palette - the Ballets Russes and Lepape's album for Poiret had not passed unnoticed - and in the more compact layout of the colour confined by the outline, now a sign of Art Deco. But Barbier's style never became completely abstract: in his White Crêpe de Chine Gown Trimmed with Fox (pl. 39) the characteristic decorative motifs of Art Deco are there but the linear rhythm still displays a suppleness reminiscent of Art Nouveau. The theme of the eighteenth century interested the young designer, as in his Longhi Masquerade (pl. 56). In his later conceptions Barbier's creative impulse showed increasing enrichment: the Black 'Charmeuse' Dress (pl. 80) and the Gala Evening Gown in Tulle and Silk (pl. 84) already show the explosions of colour and the graceful, agitated line derived from eighteenth-century art that were to characterize his work around 1920.
Bernard Boutet de Monvel was a very refined and rigorous stylist. A painter and illustrator, he contributed drawings to the Assiette au Beurre, La Vie Parisienne, Fémina, and the Gazette du Bon Ton. Poiret had taught him to design men's clothes, intending to open a fashionable shop for men, a project that never materialized. His lean, 'controlled'

style, highly abbreviated, was one of the most characteristic expressions of Art Deco.

His 'conciseness' - no doubt influenced by Cubist painting - was more suited to the creation of sober and elegant men's clothing (note his Young Gentleman's Outfit, *pl. 33*) than to clothes for women. In his creations for women, he seemed often to achieve only pallid results, devoid of invention, as in his Violet Velvet Cloak Trimmed with Natural Fox (*pl. 38*).

In Charles Martin (1848-1934), a native of Montpellier and pupil at the Académie Julian and the Atelier Cormon in Paris, there was a trace of Paul Iribe's artistic irony. He made his debut as an illustrator by contributing to Le Rire and Fémina, and later devoted himself to stage designs and interior decoration. His contributions to the Journal already show that 'amazed' look that he was to develop around 1920 (illustrations for Fantasio), and which came to be characterized by a more convulsive use of line (and by a play of juxtaposed planes derived from Cubism), here still restrained as in his White 'Crêpe' Sheath (*pl. 20*) and Crêpe de Chine Sheath (*pl. 67*).

Francisco Javier Gosé (1876-1915) was a Spanish artist who had arrived in Paris in 1900 and had been a contributor to the Assiette au Beurre since 1901. His broad and intricate style was influenced by Diaghilev's stage sets. Among the other designers, Etienne Drian and Henri Robert Dammy displayed similar linear development, and were reminiscent in their style of the sensitive line of Helleu and Chahine. Robert Pichenot occupied a position halfway between Iribe and Barbier. Valuable contributions were also made by Armand Vallée, Roger Broders and Fernand Siméon. All were sought after as designers for the best-known magazines of the time; their styles showed nineteenth-century influence, and were moderate and conciliatory expressions of the new: note the Tea Gown (*pl. 24*) by Broders, the White Velvet Tailleur (*pl. 28*) by Siméon, and the Muslin Dress (*pl. 41*) by Vallée.

Maurice Taquoy, on the other hand, a specialist in sports clothing, seemed already to foreshadow the free-and-easy manner that was later to characterize the garçonne. No. 37 (1 June 1913) carried a fine costume design by Léon Bakst for D'Annunzio's Pisanelle, in which the Russian artist confirmed his predilection for ostentation and Oriental decorative motifs. The Italian artist Umberto Brunelleschi, who was to make his name in Paris a few years later as a costume designer, was represented in No. 5 (10 July 1912) with a Walking Dress in Twilled Silk (*pl. 10*), a revival of the Empire style and distinguished by a languid line. Ismaël Smith and Aris Metzanos, among others, also designed in this vein. But did these attractive creations deserve the accolade of 'elegance'? According to Pierre Veber in No.9 (20 August 1912), there is an exacting standard to meet:

On Elegance
Elegance resides in the perfect harmony of thoughts, words, acts, gestures, attitudes, and costume.
It is through costume that elegance expresses itself most quickly.

The elegant person should not wear anything conspicuous or extreme. He refrains from colours that are too crude, clothes of eccentric cut, perfumes that are too heavy, jewelry that is too rich, excessive gestures, vocal outbursts, and words that are too strong.
The elegant person is the one who makes himself noticed by means of discretion.

'Dandyism' is not elegance, it is the exaggeration of elegance; one might also say it is the exploitation of elegance, or, if you like, the affectation of elegance.

One is born elegant, one can also become so.
It is better to be born so.

There are people whose elegance is revealed simply by a necktie.

In order to dress, one must know how to 'choose', and in order to choose, one must know oneself well. But when one knows oneself well, one must overcome the horror that one has of oneself.

The elegant woman does not launch models; she does not precede fashion, she accommodates it.

The fashions of the past are almost always ridiculous; but whatever the period, the corresponding 'elegances' are always pretty.

Ill-formed people are very often elegant; nine times out of ten, elegance is nothing but the art of taking advantage of one's flaws.

Do not say to the milliner, 'I want a pretty hat', but rather, 'I want a hat that makes me pretty'.

A young woman tells me, 'I don't care if I have ugly dresses or ugly hats. But I wouldn't wear ugly stockings or ugly shoes.'
It is fair to add that she doesn't have ugly legs.

There are hours during the day when one must not 'be dressed'. There are others when one must not 'not be dressed'.

A woman should always be ready to faint on the street.
Let us be particularly careful about 'intimate apparel'.

Avoid theatrical attire.

'I', says a newly-rich woman, 'give my old dresses to my maid. Here, at last, are some dresses that are going to be worn.

It is unusual for a well-dressed person to have mediocre thoughts. It is also unusual for him to have sublime ones.

There was a time when it was only possible for the rich to dress. This was because the dispensers of elegance were then specialists: Brummell's glove required the work of three tradesmen.

Brummel pushed elegance a little too far: so that his clothes should not be too new, he had them 'broken in' by his valet before wearing them himself. Thus Brummell's valet would say to his comrades: 'When I get tired of a coat, I give it to the master.'

An ordinary man is insolent. An elegant man is barely impertinent. Generally he is indifferent.

An elegant man is selfish. His punishment is to love an elegant woman. This rarely happens to him.

The large department stores have killed elegance. But, by the same token, they have rid us of 'dandyism': great harm in exchange for a small gain.

Cristina Nuzzi

The Artists

Léon Bakst *(Saint Petersburg 1866 - Paris 1924)*
Painter and designer. Having begun his career as a painter, he joined the Mir Iskusstva *(World of Art) group and devoted himself to stage design. In 1909 he arrived in Paris with Diaghilev's Ballets Russes. With his lively and highly colourful designs for Sheherazade (1910), the object of much discussion and scandal, he embarked on a thorough renewal of costume and set design, carried forward and completed by his successive creations for* Firebird *(1910),* Daphnis and Chloe *(1912),* Afternoon of a Faun *(1912), and* Jeux *(1913).*
Plate 73.

Georges Barbier *(Nantes 1882 - Paris 1932)*
Painter, designer, and illustrator. Studied with Jean-Paul Laurens and at the Académie des Beaux-Arts in Paris (1908-10). Became famous with two rare albums representing the dancers Nijinsky and Karsavina in the years 1913-14. A prolific illustrator, he worked for a long time in the field of theatre design, cultivating an aptitude for vivid colour effects derived from the example of Bakst. He frequently contributed to important fashion publications (Gazette du Bon Ton, Fémina, Feuillets d'Art, Vogue).
Plates 3, 8, 15, 21, 30, 35, 39, 46, 51, 56, 61, 69, 71, 80, 84, 91.

Bernard Boutet de Monvel *(Paris 1881 - Paris 1949)*
Painter, illustrator, fashion designer, and engraver. A pupil of Luc-Olivier Merson and Jean Dampt, he began his career in the first years of the century by contributing to the leading illustrated magazines of the period, such as Le Rire, L'Assiette au Beurre, Fémina, and La Vie Parisienne. At Poiret's request, he began designing fashions for men. A highly skilled designer, he contributed to such important fashion journals as the Gazette du Bon Ton, Vogue, and Harper's Bazaar, and also devoted himself to book illustration (Colonel Bramble by Maurois) and stage design.
Plates 2, 7, 16, 33, 38, 77.

Roger Broders
Plates 24, 29, 32, 36, 43.

Umberto Brunelleschi *(Montemurlo 1879 - Paris 1949)*
Painter, designer and book illustrator. After completing his studies in Florence, in 1900 he moved to Paris. In the years 1912-14 he gained esteem as a book illustrator (Contes du Temps Jadis by Perrault), and after having contributed to the leading fashion magazines of the time, he embarked on his successful career as a costume and set designer, pursued mostly in Paris (Ba-ta-clan, Les Folies-Bergère, Casino de Paris, Châtelet), but also in Italy (Teatro alla Scala), Germany, and America (Roxy Theater in New York).
Plate 10.

Louis Bureau
Interior decorator and furniture maker, fashion designer and illustrator. Was a close collaborator of Michel Dufet, who in 1913 had established a workshop for the creation of handmade furniture.
Plate 63.

H. Robert Dammy
Painter and illustrator. His delicate style shows the influence of late nineteenth-century graphics, and in particular of Eugène Grasset. Was a frequent contributor to La Vie Parisienne *and the* Gazette du Bon Ton.
Plates 48, 50, 59.

Etienne Drian
Painter, designer and illustrator. Gifted with an aptitude for a rapid, 'sketchy' style derived from Boldini and Toulouse-Lautrec. Was one of the most regular contributors to the Gazette du Bon Ton, Fémina, and Feuillets d'Art; his work was also published in Harper's Bazaar. His large decorative wall panels were exhibited at the Salons. He also illustrated books by H. de Regnier and J. Boulenger.
Plates 4, 25, 31, 62, 72.

Francisco Javier Gosé *(Lérida 1876 - Lérida 1915)*
After having studied at the Academia de las Bellas Artes in Barcelona, he arrived in Paris in 1900 where he frequented the studio of José Luis Pellicier. His drawings appeared in illustrated magazines (L'Assiette au Beurre, Le Rire), and he also contributed to Simplicissimus, the journal of political satire, before his premature death.
Plates 6, 13, 17.

Paul Iribe *(Angoulême 1883 - Menton 1935)*
Fashion designer, illustrator and decorator. Began as a cartoonist for L'Assiette au Beurre in 1901. Went on to achieve

success in various fields (fashion, theatre, interior decoration, cinema, graphics, jewelry), exerting a broad influence on taste in the years prior to the First World War. A subtle draftsman, in 1908 he executed a famous fashion album, Les robes de Paul Poiret racontées par Paul Iribe, and in 1912 supervised the decoration for the new house of Jacques Doucet, the aesthete and couturier. In 1914 he moved to America and remained there until 1930, working as a costume designer for the cinema. On his return to Paris, he created jewelry for Coco Chanel.
Plate 42.

Pierre Legrain (Levallois-Pierret 1889 - Paris 1929)
Draftsman, interior decorator, bookbinder Having studied at the Ecole des Arts Appliqués Pilon, in 1908 he became an assistant to Iribe. His drawings appeared in L'Assiette au Beurre, La Baionette, Le Temoin, and Le Mot in the years 1908-17; later, at Jacques Doucet's suggestion, he devoted himself to bookbinding, a field in which his talent was expressed more fully.
Plate 65.

Victor Lhuer
Plates 79, 89

Charles Martin (Montpellier 1848 - Montpellier 1934)
Painter, decorator, illustrator, fashion designer. After pursuing regular academic studies in his native city and Paris, he attended the Atelier Cormon. Contributed to numerous periodicals of satire and social commentary (Le Rire, Le Sourire, Fantasio) and fashion journals (Gazette du Bon Ton, Fémina, Vogue, Eve, Vanity Fair).Active in other fields as well (interior decoration and stage design), he illustrated numerous books with a dazzling satirical verve (for. T. Bernard, for Satie).
Plates 'Le choix difficile', 5, 12, 19, 20, 45, 67, 86.

Aris Metzanos
Plate 53.

Robert Pichenot
Plates 49, 54.

Lucien Robert
Painter and illustrator. Collaborator in the early years of the century on the more important satirical magazines.
Plate 70.

Fernand Siméon (1884-1928)
Painter, engraver and illustrator. Worked marginally as a

magazine contributor. while devoting himself succ... woodcuts. But his work was primarily in the field o, illustration, for texts ranging from Racine to Diderot, Gautier, and Anatole France.
Plates 18, 26, 28.

Ismaël Mari Smith (Barcelona 1886)
Sculptor, engraver and illustrator. Studied in his native city at the Academia Lonja and the Academia Baixa, and then with Atché and Carbonell. In 1910 he went to Paris on an art scholarship and attended the Ecole Nationale des Arts Décoratifs, meanwhile devoting himself to the illustration of magazines, fashion journals and books.
Plate 83.

J. Renée Souef
Illustrator and designer. She is known to have been active in 1914 as a set and costume designer for Madame Rasimi, actress-manager in revues of the time at the Ba-ta-clan.
Plate 57.

Maurice Taquoy
Painter, illustrator and engraver. In painting he depicted horses and other sporting themes. As a draftsman, with a firm and controlled line, he contributed to Fémina and La Vie Parisienne, as well as other periodicals. He exhibited at the Salon of 1905 and also devoted himself to book illustration (Le pesage by Jean Traneux).
Plates 22, 27, 47, 60.

Armand Vallée
Painter, designer and illustrator. Contributor to the leading satirical papers (Le Rire, Le Sourire, Fantasio) and fashion journals (Fémina, Modes). Worked in other fields as well (posters, stage design, book illustration).
Plates 41, 52, 55, 64, 82, 83.

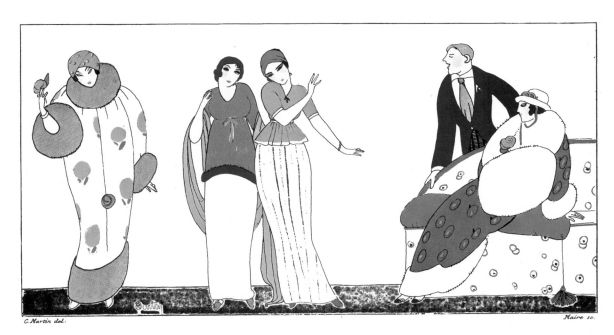

C. Martin del.   Maire sc.

LE CHOIX DIFFICILE

Dédié à l'occasion du 1er Janvier 1913 aux Amis du Journal des Dames et des Modes.

(1230)

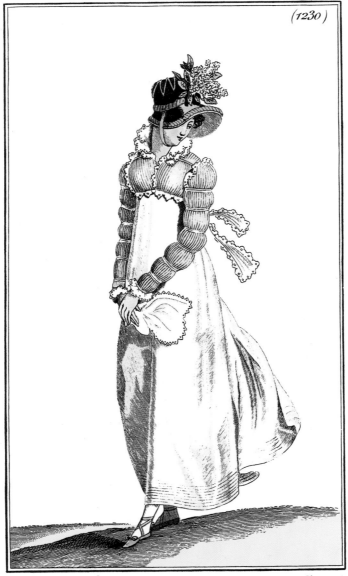

Chapeau de Gros de Naples. Canezou et Robe de Perkale

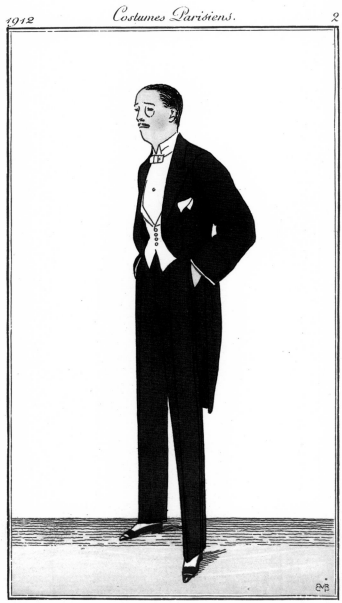

Habit de soirée. Gilet de piqué blanc. Chaussettes de soie blanche.

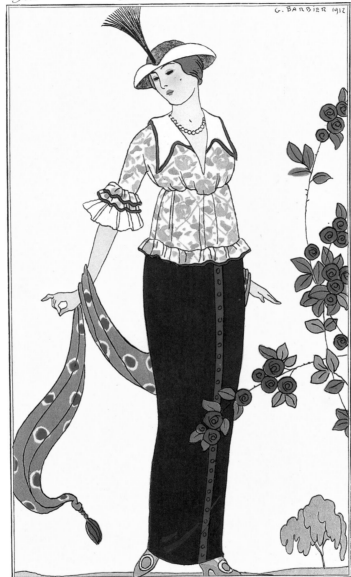

Toilette d'Été Blouse de Linon sur jupe de foulard

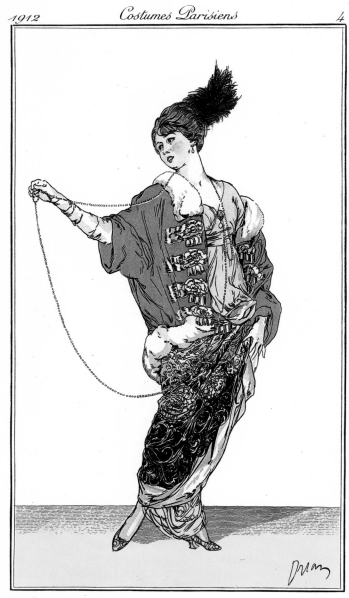

Manteau du soir en velours amarante brodé d'argent

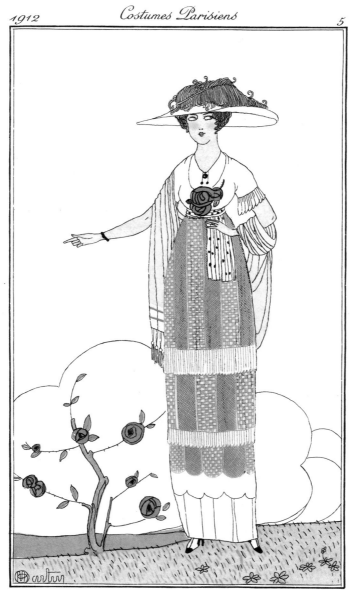

Robe de linon à haut volant de Broderie anglaise perle souliers noir et blanc

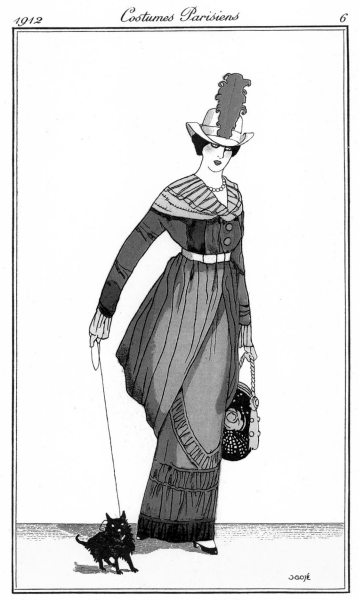

Robe à Panier en Satin café

Costume tailleur en cheviotte grise. Chemisette de Baptiste. Chapeau en paille
de riz garni Velours noir et Guêtres de Drap beige.

Tailleur de Satin gris de perle. Chapeau de paille noir

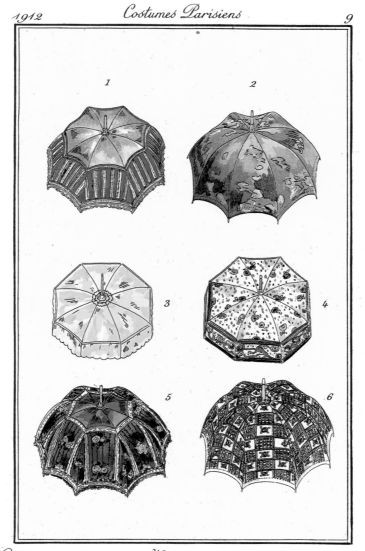

Ombrelles nouvelles: 1. en soie Kaki et cretonne imprimée pékin.-2. en Crêpe de Chine, peint à la main.-3. ombrelle de jeune fille en taffetas rose.- 4. en mousseline imprimée fond blanc.-5. en mousseline à fleurs nouvelles.-6. en cretonne imprimée à carreaux et fleurs

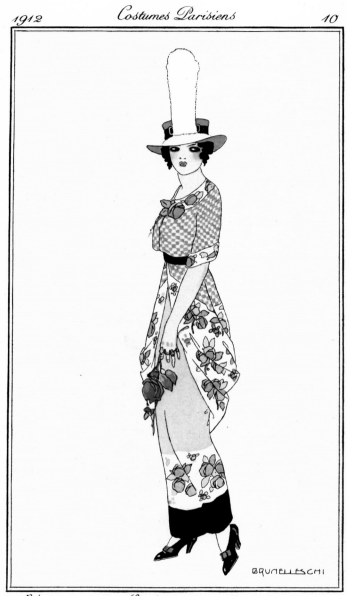

Robe de promenade en Surah à damiers et taffetas peint à la main,
bordée de velours noir. Chapeau de paille orné d'un panache en duvet de Cygne.

Robe de campagne : jaquette plissée en crêpe de Chine Évêque ;
Jupe en crêpe de Chine à fleurs.

Modèles de M.me Marcelle Demay

Chapeaux de saison : 1 en paille d'Italie, passe velours, garni Paradis ; 2, toque de satin garni d'aigrettes ; 3, en tagal blanc, garni roses et feuillage ; 4, en paille d'Italie, fleurs des champs ; 5 en tulle blanc, roses et crosse ; 6 en feutre blanc, garni peau de Suède ; 7 en paille d'Italie, couteaux autruche ; 8 panama et mousseline imprimée ; 9, en crêpe crêpé blanc, garni paradis ; 10, en mousseline garni autruches et roses.

Fourreau de satin noir ouvert sur intérieur de linon blanc plissé.
Chapeau en peau de soie noire avec garniture blanche.

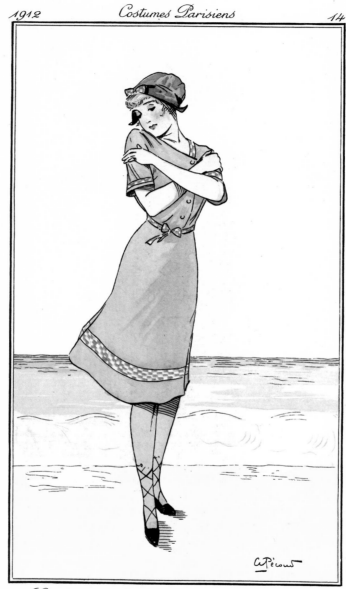

Costume de bain en taffetas changeant

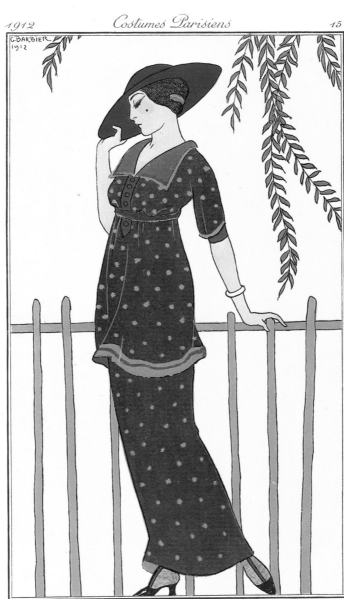

Robe de plage en foulard garni de tussor gros grain chapeau en Suède rouge

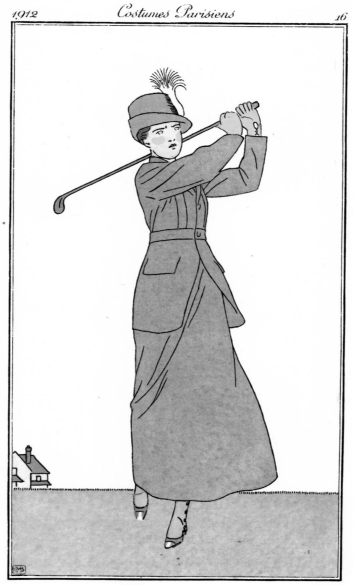

Blouse à plis creux en toile Kaki guêtres hautes en drap beige chapeau de feutre

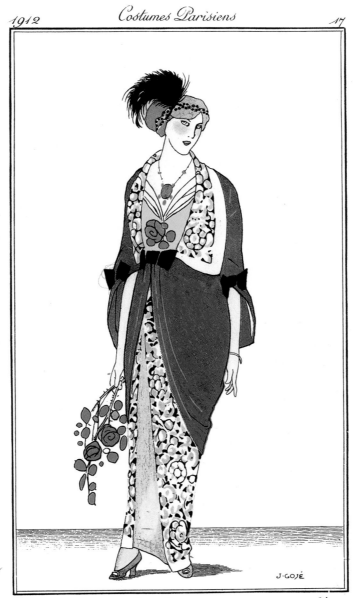

J·GOJÉ

Manteau du soir en Satin bleu cendre avec garnitures d'Irlande

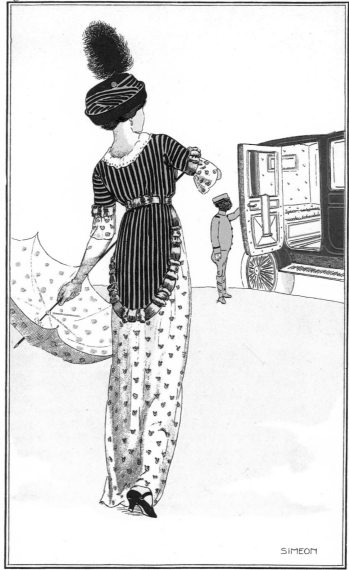

Veste de velours pékiné noir et auburn sur fourreau de frissonnette peinte. — Chapeau velours et aigrette

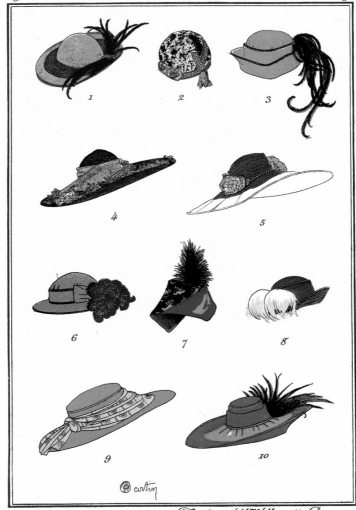

— Modèles de Mme Marcelle Demay

Chapeaux d'Automne : 1. Satin blanc, fantaisie Paradis noir. 2. Bonnet Hollandais, fond or broderie laine couleurs 3. Tricorne velours et Paradis olive. 4. En velours et moire, couronne d'autruche frisée. 5. Bergère Louis XVI, crêpe de Chine blanc, panne noire et camelias 6. velours canard pouff autruche. 7. Bonnet du soir, broché, œuf d'aigrette. 8 Le Mignon : en velours noir, boules multifil. 9. En velours saphir, soierie écossaise 10. en velours fantaisie Paradis rubis.

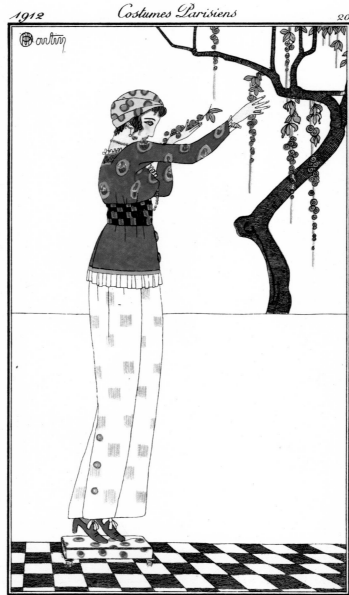

Fourreau crépe blanc brodé et peint. Blouse velours
émeraude broché ponceau. Ceinture de perles.

Robe de drap blanc bordé d'un ourlet couleur de rose.
Ceinture de roses au crochet

Costume de chasse en laine d'Écosse

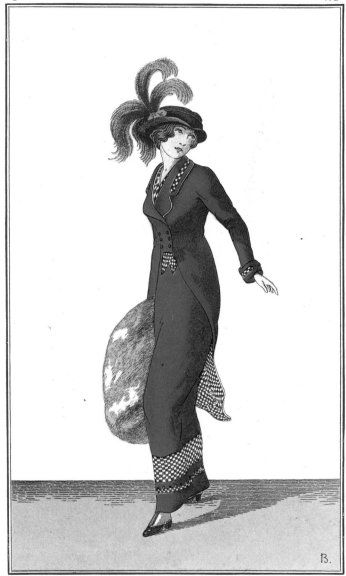

Robe en velours de laine bleu avec longue jaquette de même étoffe
doublée et garnie de velours à petit damier

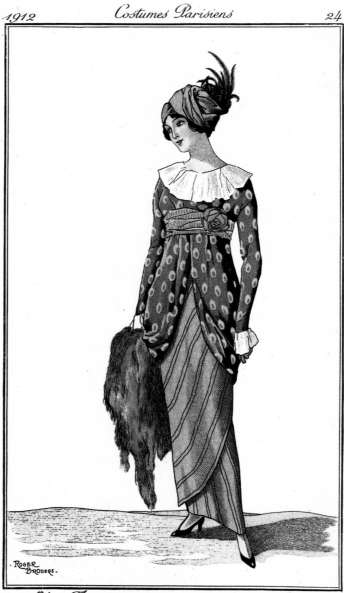

Robe de Thé en velours aubergine ocellé d'œils de Paon
Fourreau gris d'Acier. Turban aigretté d'un Lophophore

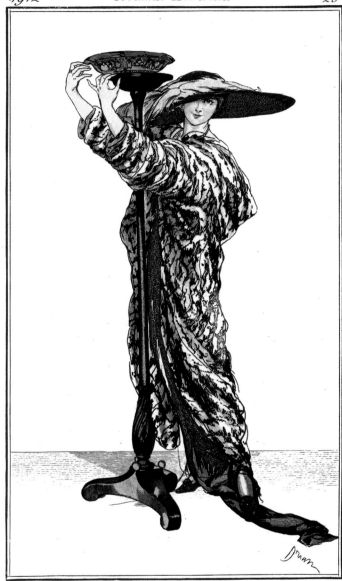

Grand Manteau de Chinchilla

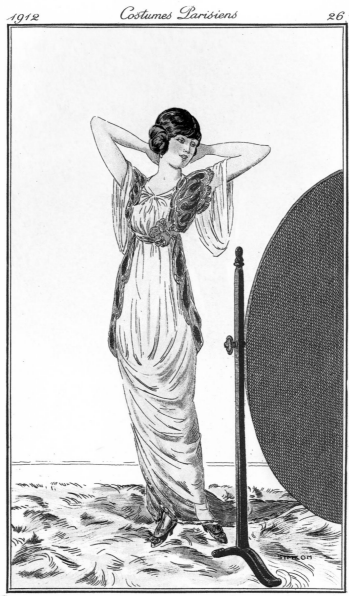

Deshabillé de mousseline de soie glycine drapé et bordé de fourrure.
Petite casaque de velours noir frappé.

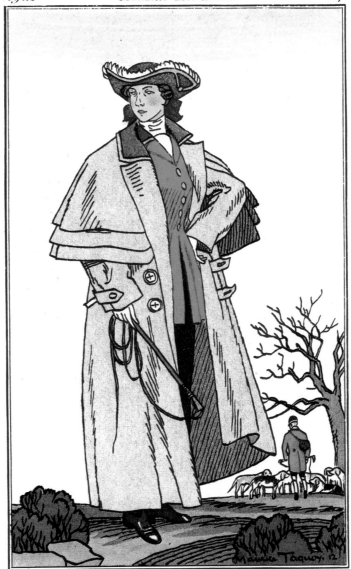

Tenue d'Équipage. Carrik en drap souris

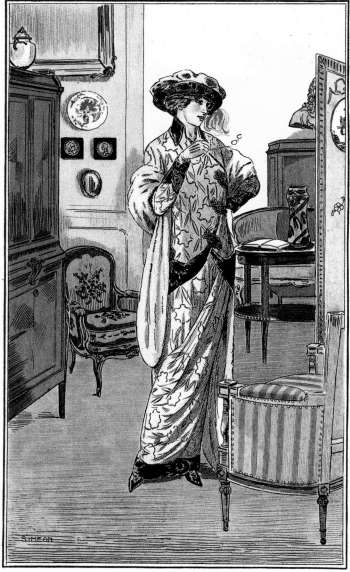

Tailleur de Velours blanc frappé
garni de Loutre et de Passementerie

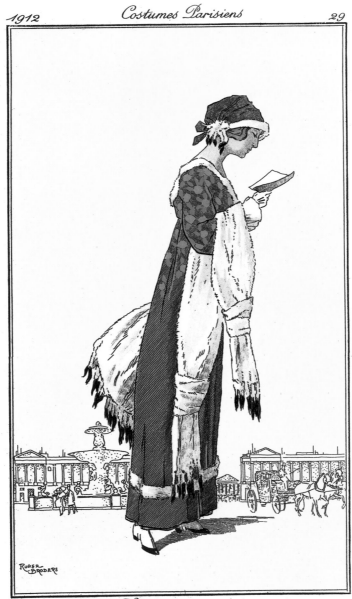

Robe et Toque de velours de soie
vert de mer bordées d'hermine

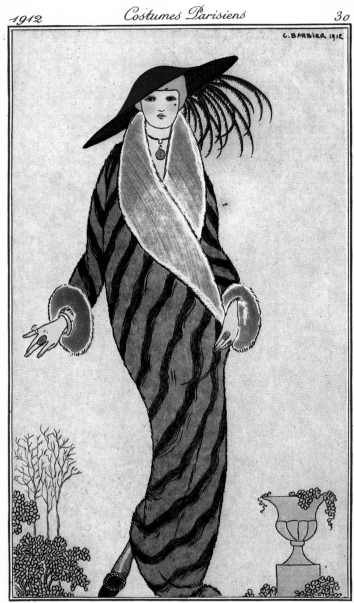

Manteau de Zibeline à col et poignets de renard blanc

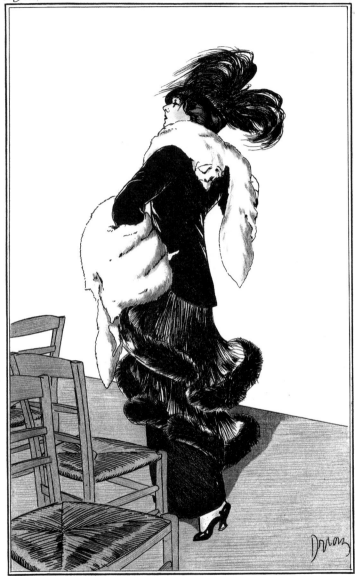

*Robe de velours à double tunique de mousseline de soie
bordée de skunks: Étole et manchon de renard blanc.*

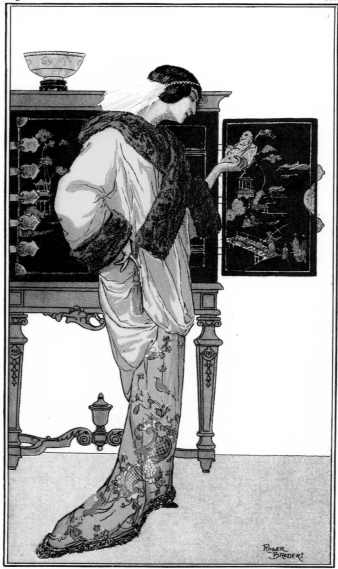

*Robe de soie de Chine bordée de Chinchilla. Manteau de velours
citron vert à grand Col et parements de Chinchilla, gland d'Argent*

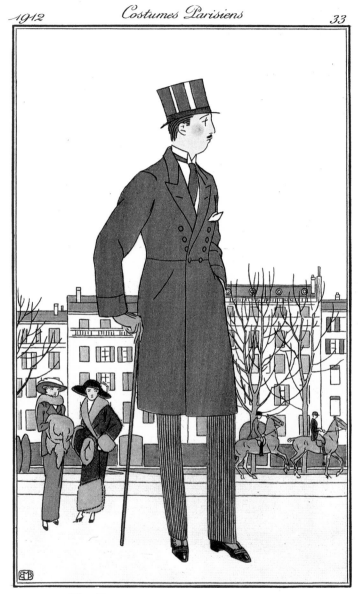

Mise d'un jeune homme

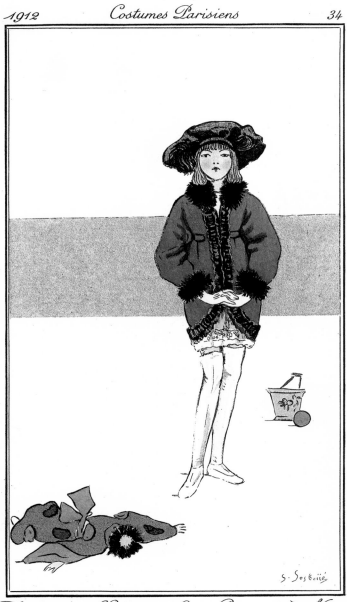

Manteau de fillette en velours bleu garni de Skungs
Guêtres de Suède blanc

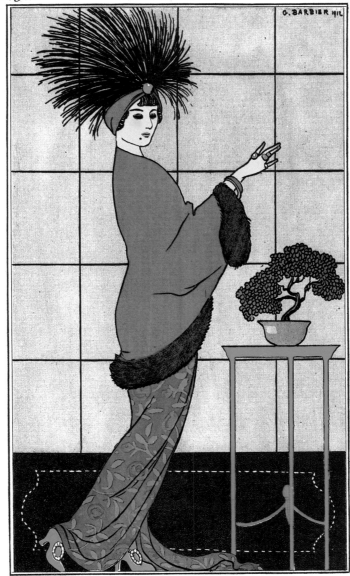

Manteau de Damas rose garni de Renard bleu
Coiffure de Paradis noirs

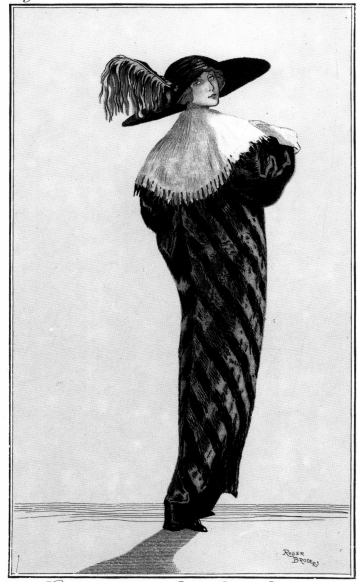

Grand manteau de Loutre. Col d'hermine
Chapeau noir à plume changeante

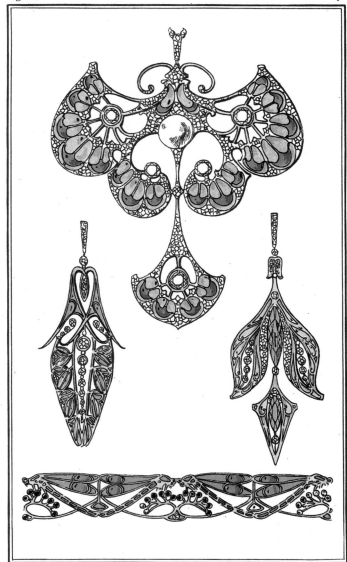

Bijoux par Veyer
Pendants de cou joaillerie et émaux translucides
Bracelet libellules émaux et diamants.

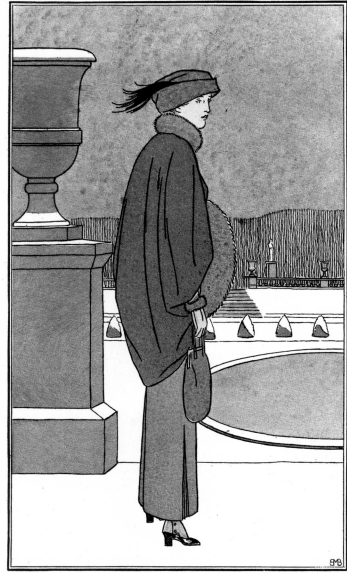

Manteau de velours violet garni de renard naturel
Tailleur de drap vert verre.

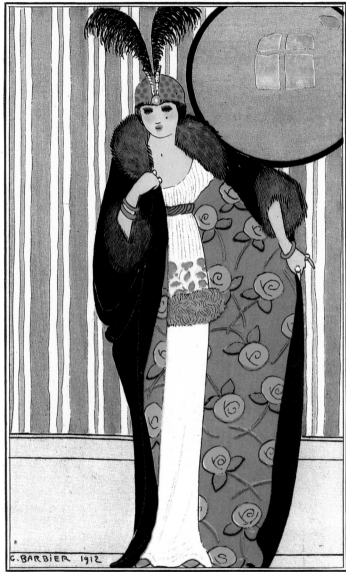

Robe de crêpe de Chine blanc garnie de renard
Manteau de loutre et skunks

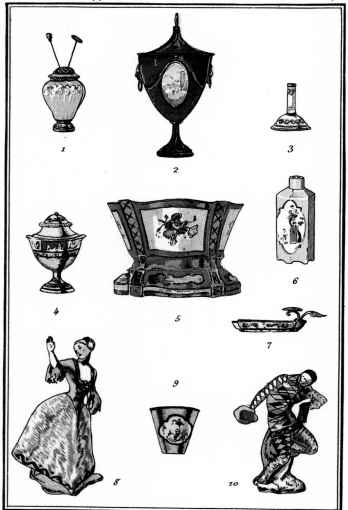

Modèles de Géo Rouard "A la Paix"
1. Porte-épingles à chapeau en porcelaine tendre montée
bronze 2-9. Vernis-Martin. 3-4-5-6. Vases , Jardinière,
et boîte à thé en pâte tendre 7. Cendrier émail ancien
8-10. Figurines de Saxe et de Nymphenburg.

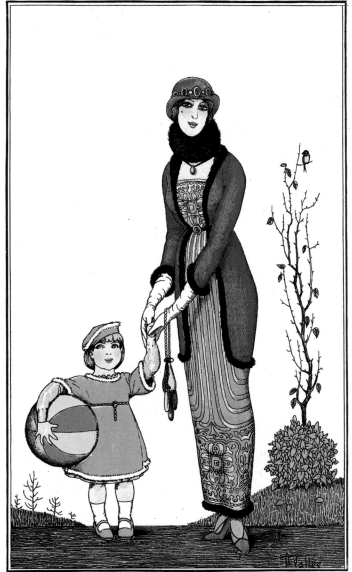

Robe de Mousseline de soie brodée et soutachée, à jaquette ouverte bordée
de Skungs. — Costume d'enfant en Ottoman corail rose bordé de Cygne.

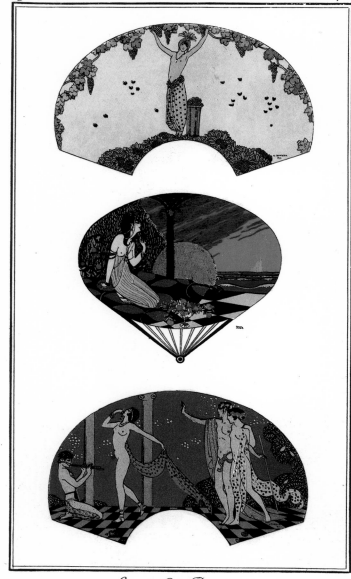

Eventails de Paquin
d'après G. Barbier et Paul Iribe

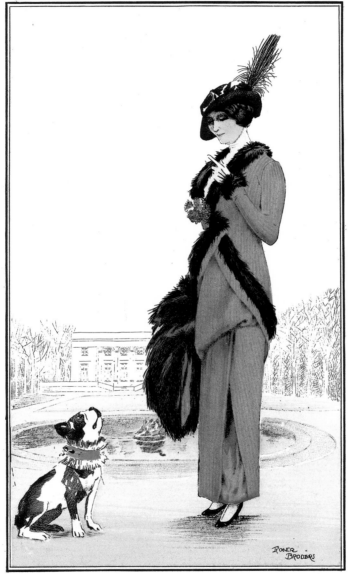

Tailleur du matin en velours de laine orné de Skungs

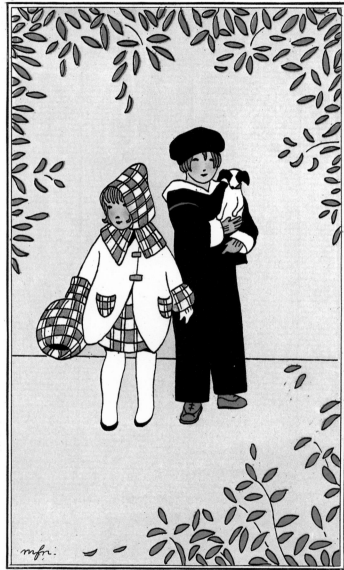

Manteau de ratine blanche, garniture écossaise jaune et blanc.
Marin blanc et noir, fox blanc et noir

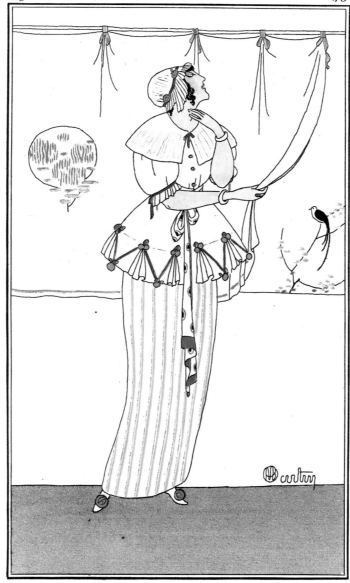

Deshabillé du matin

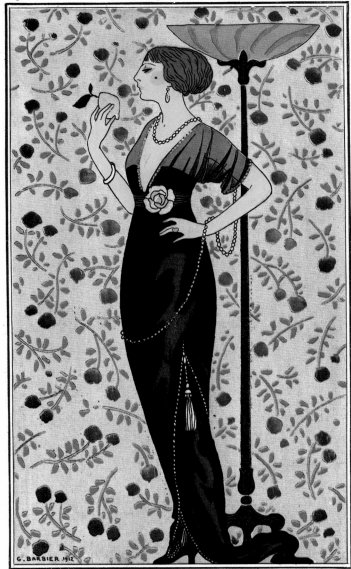

Robe du soir, satin noir et tulle, bordée de brillants.

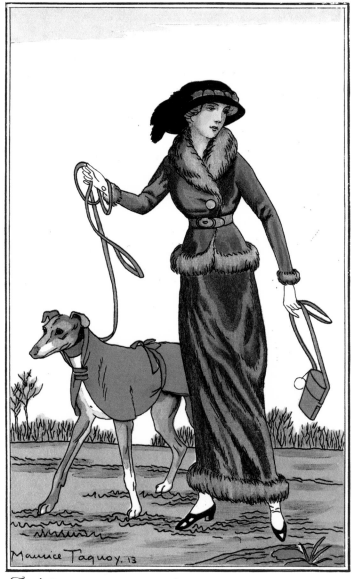

Toilette de coursing en velours prune, garnie d'opossum,
souliers de chasse à guêtres blanches.

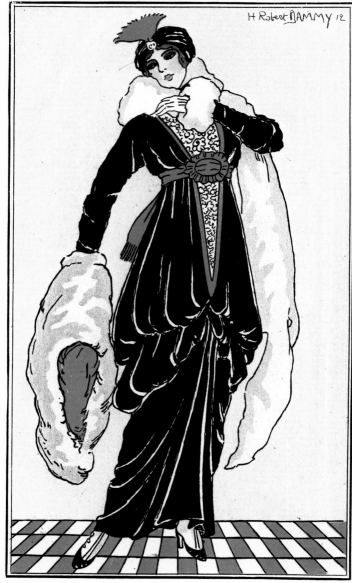

Robe d'après-midi en velours noir et satin vert.

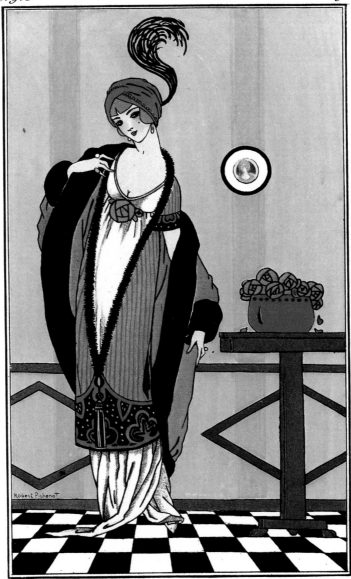

Robe de charmeuse blanche à tunique de mousseline de soie violette
brodée de vert et bordée de skungs. Manteau de velours étrusque.

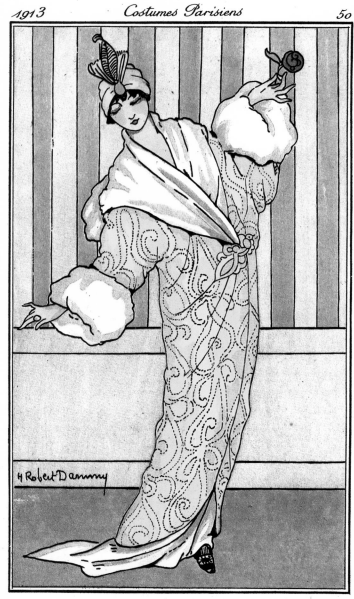

Manteau de velours frappé citron. Col velours blanc et Renard blanc.

Pour St Moritz. Ratine blanche garnie de Skunks et brodée de laines.

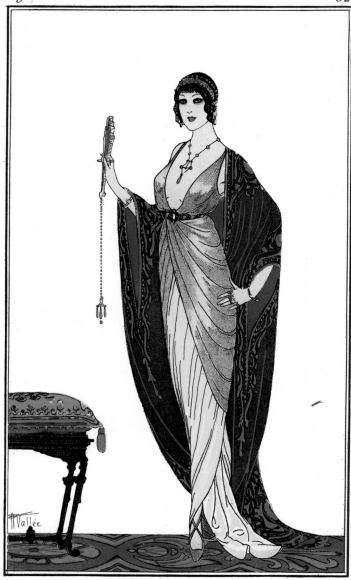

Grande Parure

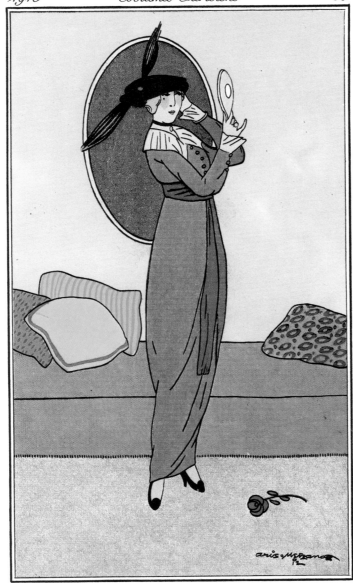

Toilette d'après Midi

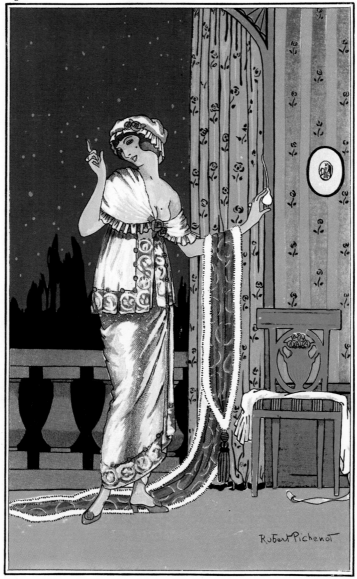

Toilette de Nuit en linon à pois garnie de dentelle et de petites roses.

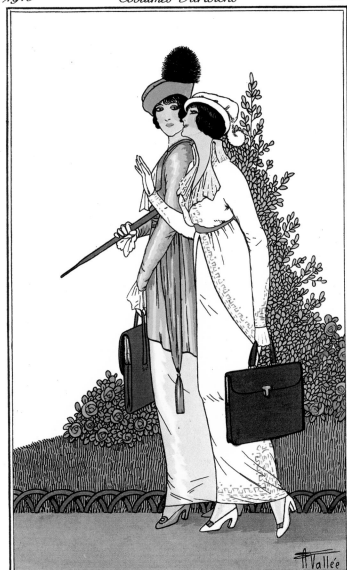

Robes de jeunes filles : l'une en crépon blanc et taffetas
orange ; l'autre en drap blanc brodé.

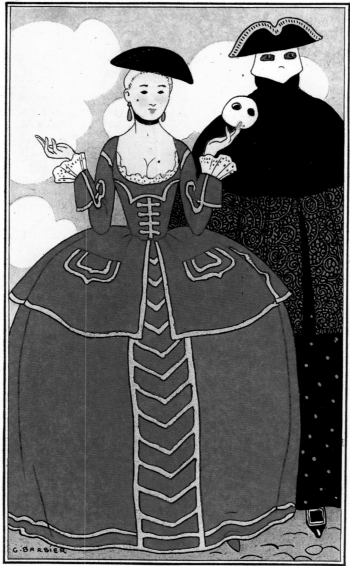

*Travestissement d'après Longhi: Robe de damas galonnée de blanc
sur laquelle on jettera une baüte de taffetas noir et de dentelle*

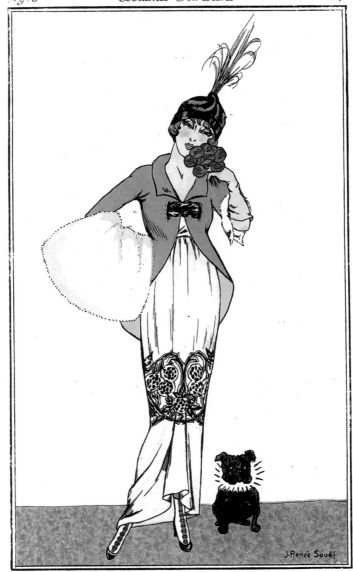

Robe de cachemire de soie brodé au passé. Jaquette de
velours de laine doublée de satin jonquille.

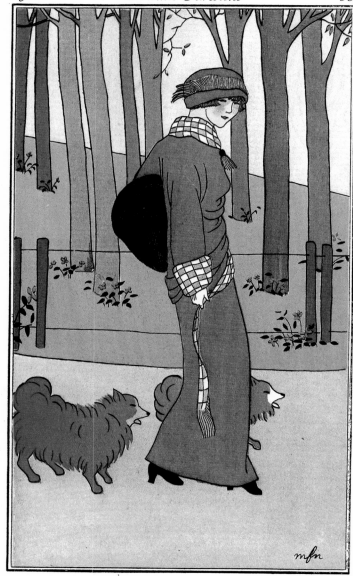

*Costume tailleur du matin en lainage vert-de-gris, ceinture
parements et col en taffetas écossais jaune et gris.*

Robe de jeune fille en crêpe de chine Blanc et garnie de velours noirs

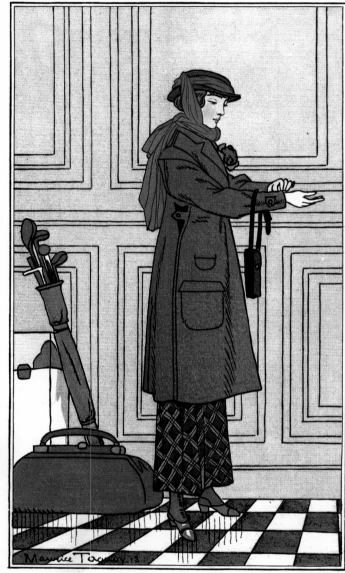

Petit loden Tailleur en laine d'Écosse . Grosses bottines lacées

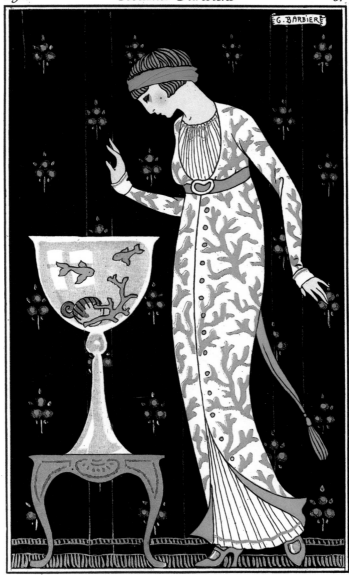

Robe d'intérieur en soie brochée, ouverte sur un dessous de linon.

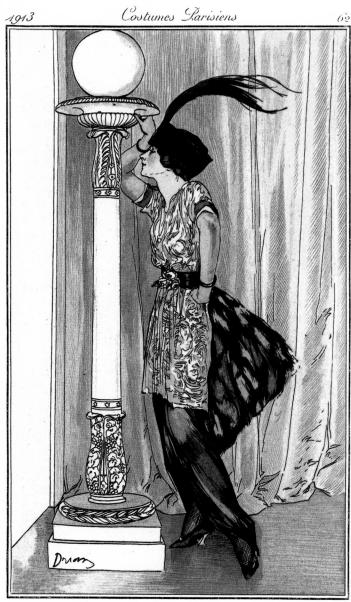

Tunique de Mousseline vieil or brodée
Manchon de Léopard

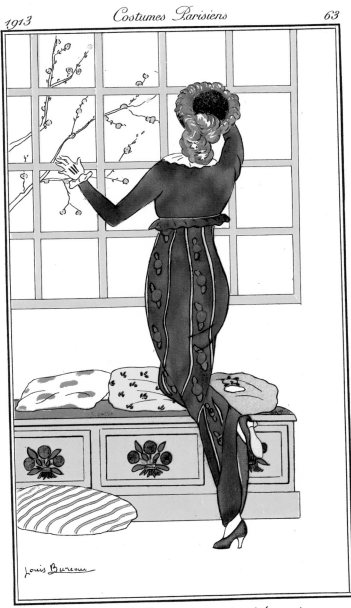

Robe de voile bleu ancien peint à la main

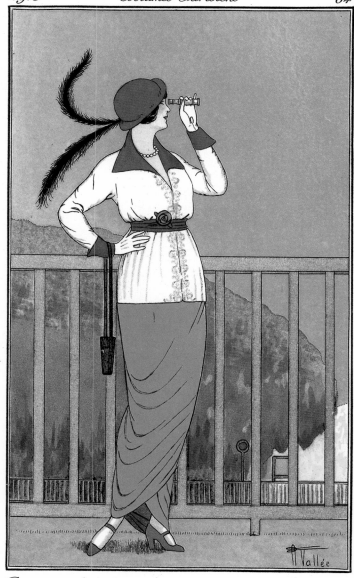

Blouse de satin blanc brodée. Jupe drapée de cachemire de soie

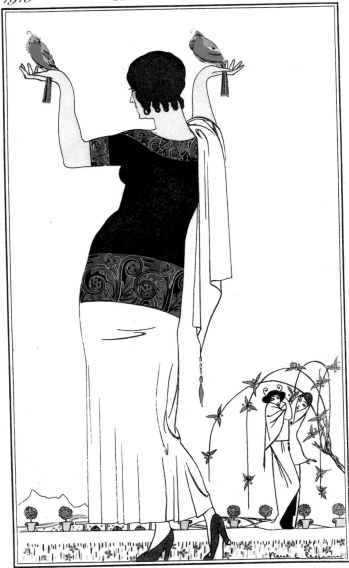

Robe d'Intérieur

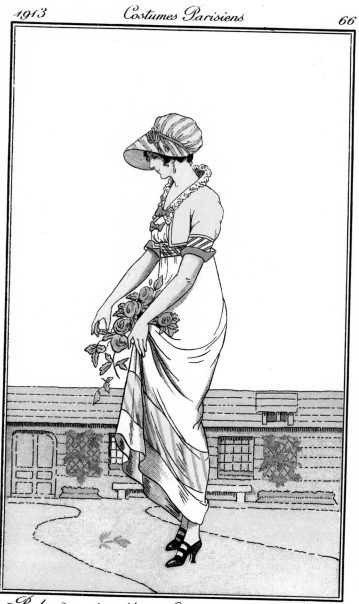

Robe de crépon blanc — Casaque de taffetas soufre —
Bonnet de taffetas pékiné.

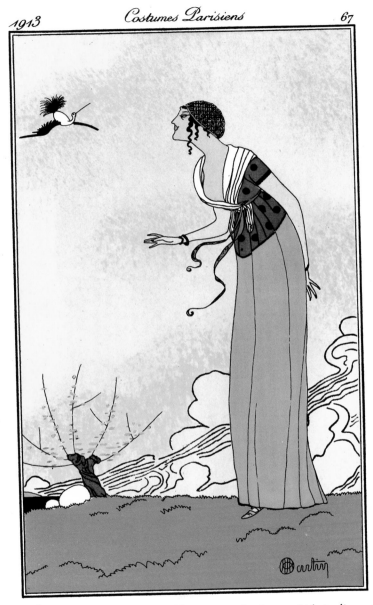

Fourreau de crêpe de Chine - Veste de satin brodée à châle de linon

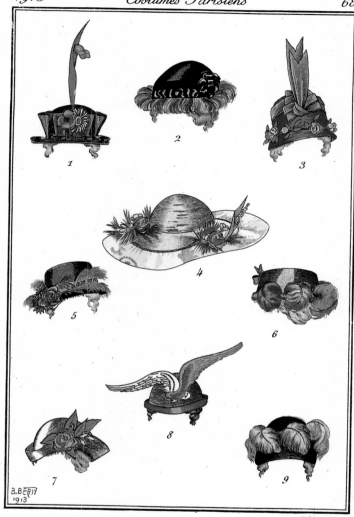

Modèles de Marcelle Demay

1, 2, 4, 6: le Bronzino - le Peau-d'Âne, le Berri & le Beaujolais: en picot, garnitures de plumes et de fleurs. 3, 5, 8, 9: la Roseraie, l'Ophélie, la Walkyrie & le Consort: en tagal, garnitures de rubans, mousseline, fleurs, plumes & ailes fantaisie. 7: le Delmar, en paille garni de feuillages.

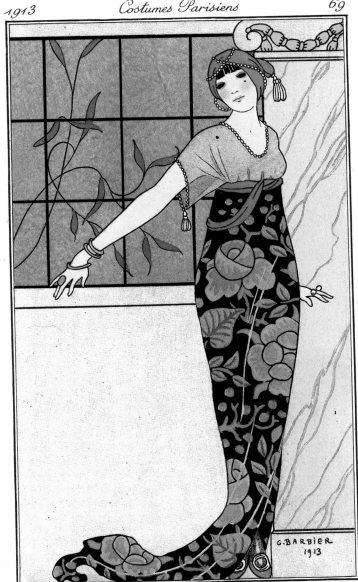

Grande robe du soir, corsage de mousseline chair, tunique de soie
brodée dans le goût de la "Compagnie des Indes".

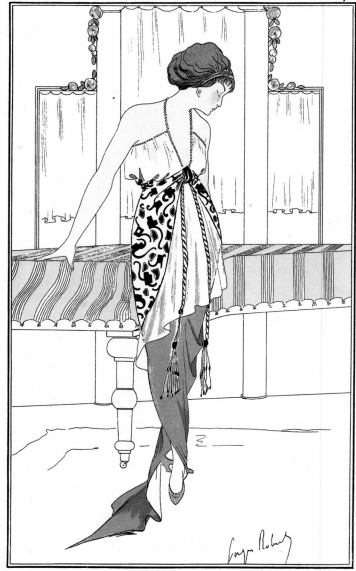

*Robe de satin bleu recouverte d'une tunique de tulle blanc
sur laquelle se drape un brocart de Chine noir et blanc.*

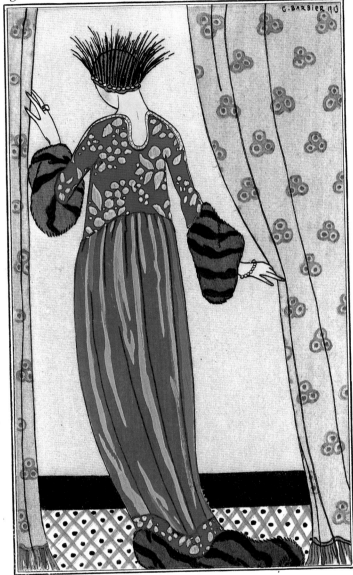

Manteau de Théâtre

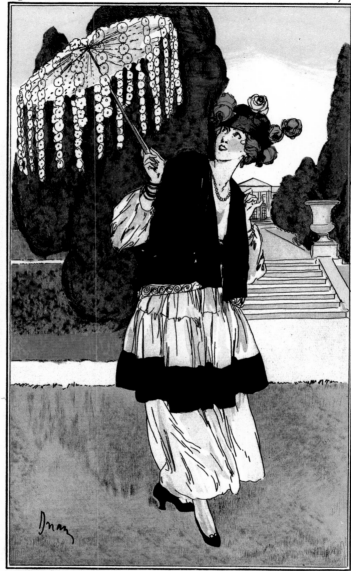

Robe de mousseline de soie à volant bordé de satin noir.
Casaque vague aussi de satin noir.

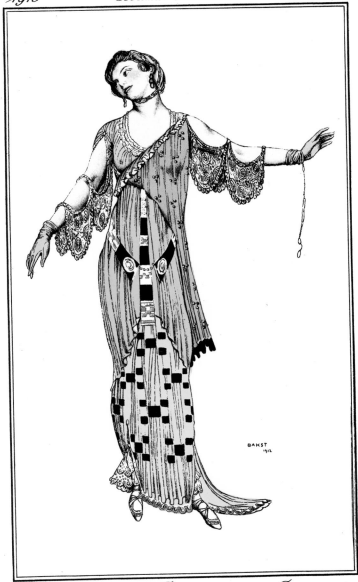

Dioné.- dessin de Bakst réalisé par Paquin.

1.2.3. Porcelaines de la Manufacture Royale de Saxe.— 4.5.6.—
pâte tendre de Mennecy.—8.10. Manufacture Royale de Nymphenbourg.—
7 et 9. Faïences de Wedgwood. (Se trouvent chez Géo Rouard, "A la Paix".)

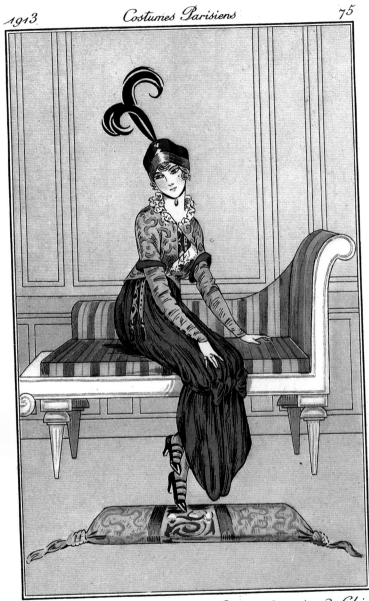

Jupe de mousseline de soie marine. Casaque de Crêpe de Chine
broché turquoise rehaussé de broderies rubis

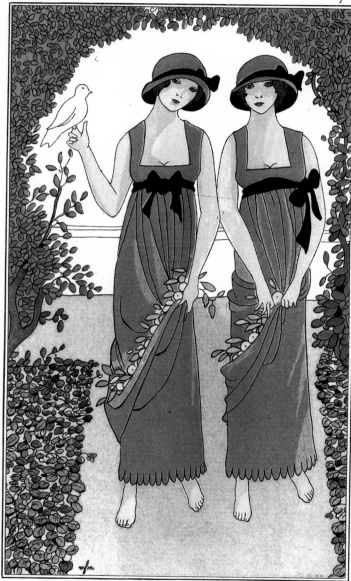

Robe de jardin en toile bleu vif, ceinture de velours noir.— Chapeau toile et velours.

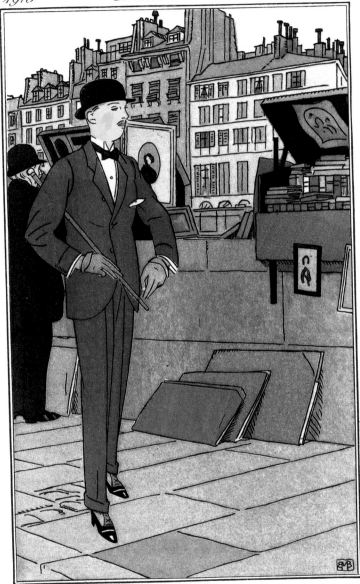

Tenue du matin

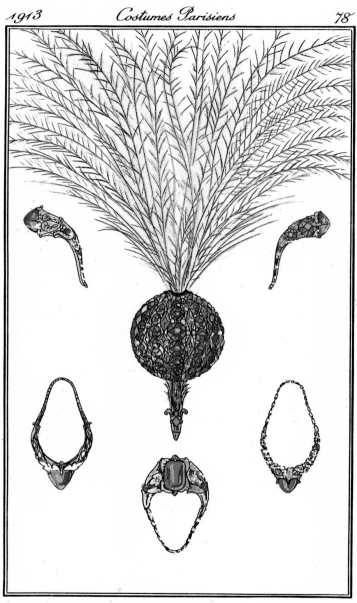

Aigrette et bagues souples par Morgan.

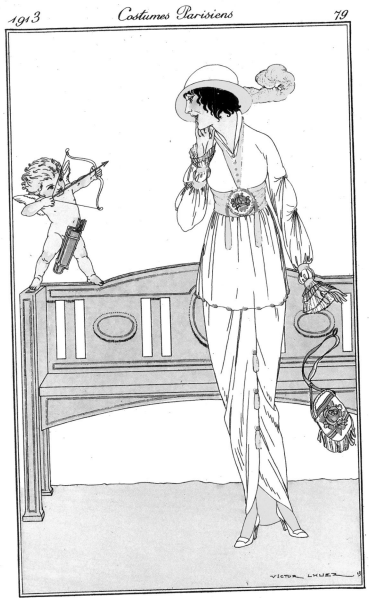

Robe de crêpe de Chine._ Sac et ceinture brodés de perles.

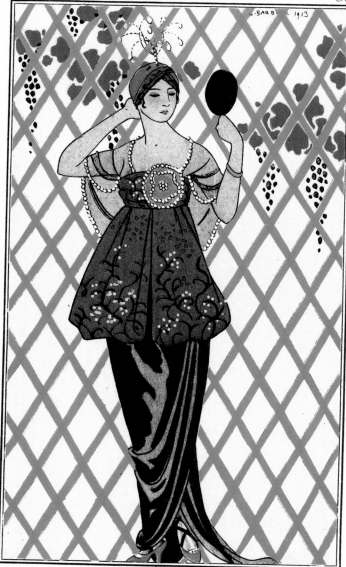

*Robe de charmeuse noire avec corsage et panier
formés d'un obi drapé.*

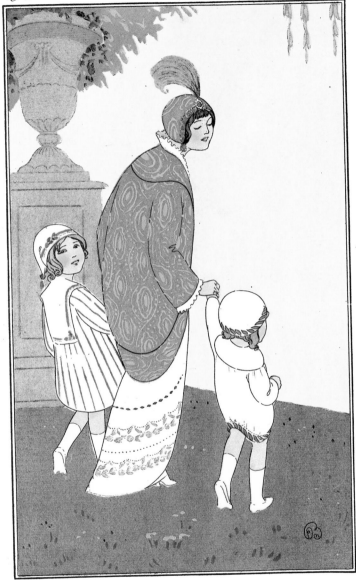

Toilettes de promenade

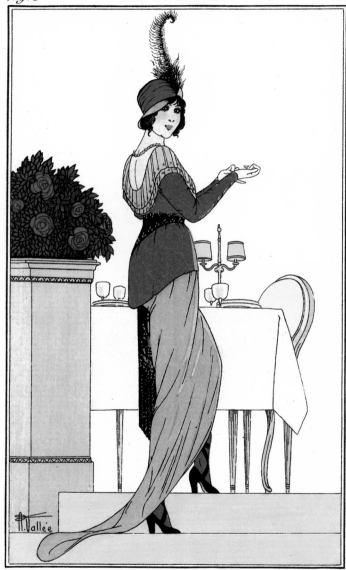

Robe pour dîner au Bois.

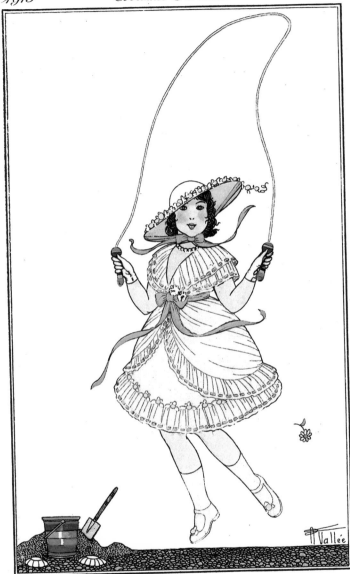

Costume d'une Demoiselle de 6 à 8 ans.

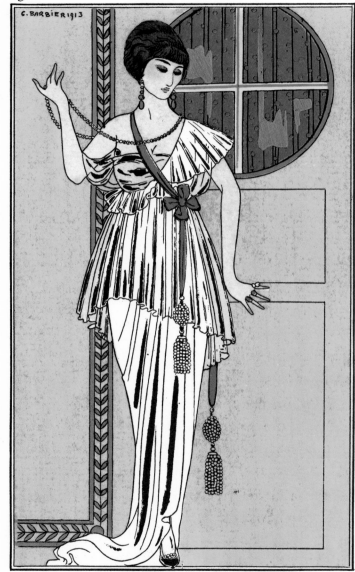

Grande robe du soir en tulle et satin. —
Écharpe de velours à glands de perles.

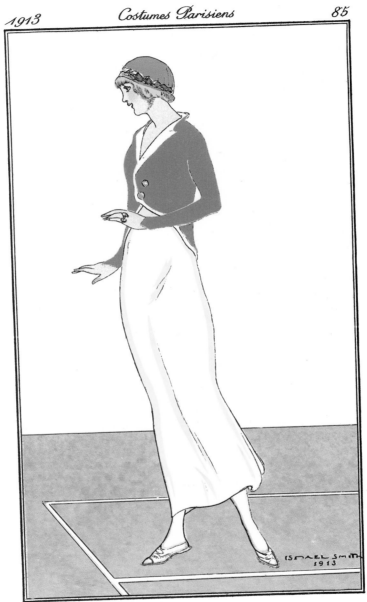

Costume de tennis

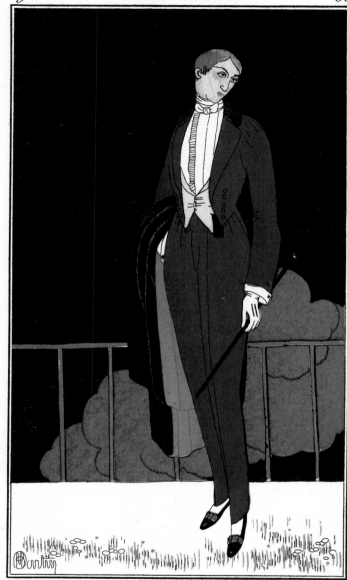

Habit nouveau par Kriegck

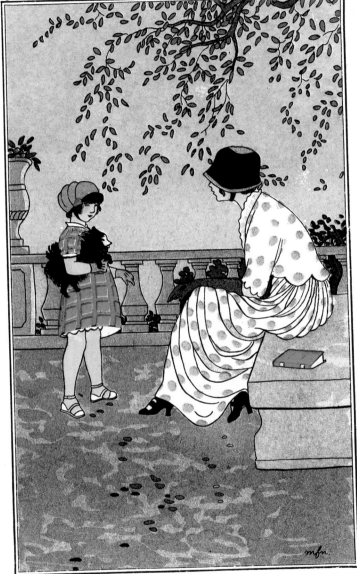

Robe de crépon blanc à pois jaune. — Robe de fillette
en écossais cerise et vert.

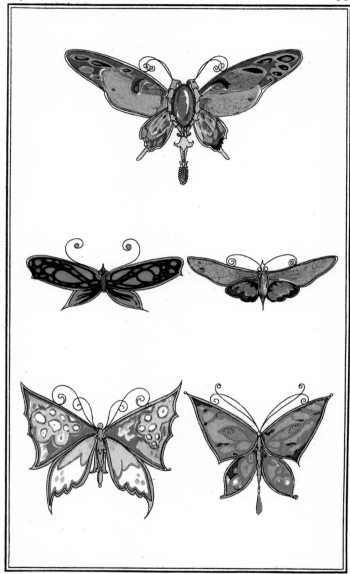

Papillons naturels montés en diamants par Morgan.

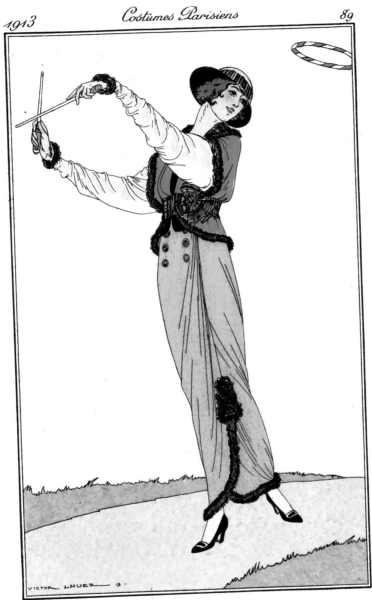

Toilette de garden-party

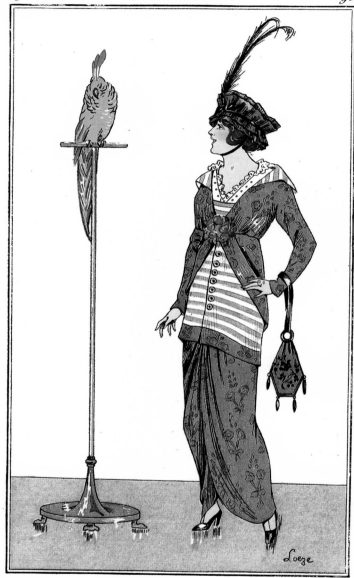

Robe de taffetas à fleurs et ottoman de soie.—Chapeau de tulle.

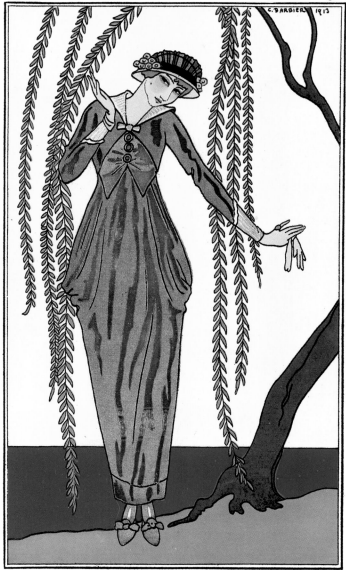

Robe de taffetas gris à col et manchettes de linon
et gilet de satin à boutons d'émail.

Gants de Suède et de chevreau glacé